Anissa Zaouak
Houda Hammami
Samy Fenniche

# Acute generalized exanthematous pustulosis

**Anissa Zaouak**
**Houda Hammami**
**Samy Fenniche**

# Acute generalized exanthematous pustulosis

## Toxidermia

**ScienciaScripts**

**Imprint**

Any brand names and product names mentioned in this book are subject to trademark, brand or patent protection and are trademarks or registered trademarks of their respective holders. The use of brand names, product names, common names, trade names, product descriptions etc. even without a particular marking in this work is in no way to be construed to mean that such names may be regarded as unrestricted in respect of trademark and brand protection legislation and could thus be used by anyone.

Cover image: www.ingimage.com

This book is a translation from the original published under ISBN 978-620-6-72092-8.

Publisher:
Sciencia Scripts
is a trademark of
Dodo Books Indian Ocean Ltd. and OmniScriptum S.R.L publishing group

120 High Road, East Finchley, London, N2 9ED, United Kingdom
Str. Armeneasca 28/1, office 1, Chisinau MD-2012, Republic of Moldova, Europe
Printed at: see last page
**ISBN: 978-620-8-04195-3**

# TABLE OF CONTENTS

# INTRODUCTION

Acute generalised exanthematous pustulosis (AGEP) is a rare toxidermia and is one of the serious or severe cutaneous adverse drug reactions (SCAR). It is an erythematous, edematous and putular febrile cutaneous reaction, most often caused by drugs. It may also be due to a viral infection (enterovirus: coxsackie, echovirus or cytomegalovirus), a toxic substance (mercury) or a food allergen [1]. All ages are affected. The drugs most often responsible are antibiotics such as beta-lactams and pristinamycin [2-7]. PEAG is a model of delayed drug hypersensitivity mediated by CD8 T lymphocytes [3,4]. The onset of this toxidermia is short, ranging from a few hours to a few days [2]. Diagnosis of this dermatosis is based on clinical and paraclinical criteria. These criteria were validated by a score established in 2001 by the European SCAR study group (EuroSCAR) [4]. Clinically, PEAG manifests as a bright red, sometimes scarlatiniform, oedematous erythema covering the trunk, limbs, and particularly the axillary and inguinal folds. The rash is often accompanied by hyperthermia and neutrophilic leukocytosis [4-6,8-11].This rare skin reaction is clinically severe and may be confused with other skin reactions that can lead to the appearance of pustules, such as generalised pustular psoriasis, pustular vasculitis, drug hypersensitivity syndrome (DRESS syndrome), Lyell's syndrome and epidermal toxic necrolysis.Recovery is rapid, in one to two weeks, without any specific treatment, often following discontinuation of the drug responsible. [4-6,13]. The prognosis for this type of toxidermia is often good [4,13,14]. Few Tunisian studies have focused on this rare and potentially severe dermatosis, hence the interest of this retrospective, monocentric, descriptive study conducted at the Dermatology Department of the Habib Thameur Hospital in Tunis over 14 years (January 2008-December 2021). The aim of this study is to examine the epidemiological, clinical, therapeutic and evolutionary characteristics of drug-induced acute generalised exanthematous pustulosis.

# METHODS

## 1. Type of study

This is a retrospective descriptive study of all cases of acute generalized exanthematous pustulosis followed up at the Dermatology Department of Habib Thameur Hospital in Tunis over a 14-year period from January 2008 to December 2021.

## 2. Population of the study

### 2.1. Inclusion criteria :

During the study period, 30 cases of suspected PEAG were investigated. collected. We included in our study all cases meeting the diagnostic criteria for PEAG established by the EuroSCAR study group for suspected PEAG.

### 2.2. Non-inclusion criteria

We did not include patients who had an erythematous-pustular rash secondary to another cause.

**Table I:** Revised PEAG criteria according to study group EuroSCAR [4,5]

| Skin lesions | |
| --- | --- |
| Pustules | Typical* +2 |
| | Compatible** +1 |
| | Not assessable*** 0 |
| Erythema | Typical* +2 |
| | Compatible** +1 |
| | Not assessable*** 0 |

| | |
|---|---|
| Distribution | Typical* +2 |
| | Compatible** +1 |
| | Non-assessable*** (*)    0 |
| Post-pustular desquamation | Yes    +1 |
| | No or not assessable 0 |
| Other signs | |
| Mucosal damage | Yes-2 |
| Sudden onset <10 days | No    0 |
| | Yes    0 |
| | No. 2 |
| Cure < 15 days | Yes    0 |
| Fever > 38°C | No. 2 |
| | Yes    +1 |
| PNN > 7000 elements/mm3 | No    0 |
| | Yes    +1 |
| | No    0 |
| Histology | |
| Other illness | -10 |
| Non-representative or no biopsy | 0 |
| Exocytosis of neutrophils | +1 |
| Non-spongiform pustule, with oedema From papillary dermis or spongiform pustule without oedema of the dermis | +2 |
| Spongiform pustule with oedema of the papillary dermis | +3 |

*typical: A dozen small pustules less than 5 mm in diameter, not follicular.

** compatible: non-typical pustules that do not strongly suggest another diagnosis.

*** not assessable: aspect cannot be judged [late stage of the disease].

The score obtained by using this table is interpreted as follows Score ≤ 0: Case not considered a PEAG case. Score between 1 and 4: PEAG possible. Score between 5 and 7: probable PEAG. Score between 8 and 12: PEAG certain.

## 2.2. Exclusion criteria

We have excluded :

- Dossiers with missing information that cannot be used to calculate the EuroSCAR score.

- Patients with a EuroSCAR score of less than 1.

## 3. Collection of data

The investigative tool used in the study was a pre-established information sheet in which epidemiological, clinical, para-clinical, therapeutic and evolutionary data were recorded. This information was collected from the patients' medical records.

## 3.1. Epidemiological data

- The patient's age, sex and address.

- Personal history:

- Medical: atopy, drug allergies

- Surgical

- Family history

## 3.2. Data

- The history of the disease, the mode of onset and the duration of the course of symptomatology

- Chronology of onset of skin signs in relation to drug intake

- First episode or recurrence.

### 3.3. Examination data physical

- General signs: general condition, temperature, state of hydration, etc.

- Skin signs: elementary lesions (pustules, macules, erosions),

..., the number of lesions and their topography.

- Pleuropulmonary signs: respiratory rhythm, presence of

rales...

- Cardiovascular signs: heart rate, blood pressure, etc.

- Abdominal signs: hepatomegaly, splenomegaly, etc.
- Joint or muscle signs

### 3.4. Data from specialist consultations :

- Pharmacovigilance consultation

### 3.5. Paraclinical data :

Biological tests :

- Blood count (CBC)

- Speed of sedimentation (SV), C Reactive Protein (CRP), fibrinogen, protein electrophoresis (EPP).

- Transaminases (ASAT/ALAT), Phosphatase alkaline (PAL), Gammaglutamyltransferase ($\gamma$GT), Total and direct bilirubin.

- Blood ionogram, creatinine.

- X-ray examinations: chest X-ray.

## 3.6. Anatomopathological study :

Histopathological examination of the lesions reveals intraepidermal and/or subcorneal pustules, often multilocular and spongiform, associated with oedema of the dermal papilla with an infiltrate of neutrophils and, less frequently, eosinophils (one third of patients).

## 3.7. Data from the pharmacovigilance survey: drug imputability score :

In our study and in pharmacovigilance investigations carried out by the national pharmacovigilance centre, drug imputability is assessed by the Bégaud score (French method of drug imputability) [16].

## 3.8. Therapeutic data :

Local treatments: soothing creams, dermocorticoids.

Systemic treatments: systemic corticosteroids.

## 3.9. Evolution :

Length of follow-up after diagnosis.

Course: recurrence, cure, progression to pustular psoriasis.

## 4. Computer hardware and statistical analysis :

The data for our study were entered using Excel 2010 and analysed using SPSS 20.

## 5. Bibliographical research :

We used the following search engines for this research: PubMed and Google Scholar and the Science direct, clinicalkey and Embase websites. The keywords used were : Pustulosis, exanthematous, acute, generalised, toxidermia.

## 6. Ethical considerations and conflict of interest :

We have no conflicts of interest to declare. During the course of this work, anonymity was respected to avoid any ethical problems.

**RESULTS**

## 1. Epidemiology :

### 1.1. Impact :

The incidence of acute generalised exanthematous pustulosis was estimated at 0.9 cases/10000 consultants in our department/year.

### 1.2. Age :

In our study, the mean age was 44.7 years, with extremes ranging from from 7 to 85 years old.

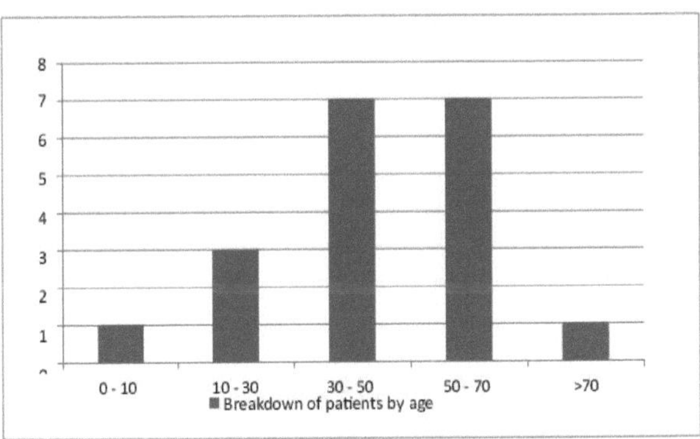


**Figure 1:** Age distribution of patients

### 1.3. Gender :

In our study, the patients were divided into 15 women and 4 men, giving an M/F sex ratio of 0.26.

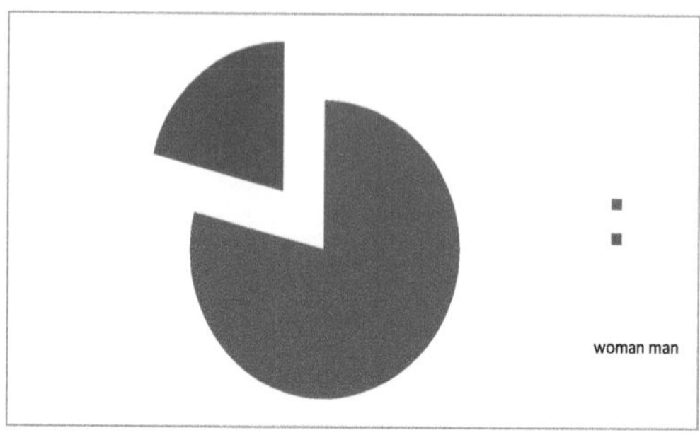


**Figure 2:** Breakdown of patients by gender

## 1.4. Breakdown of patients by age and sex :

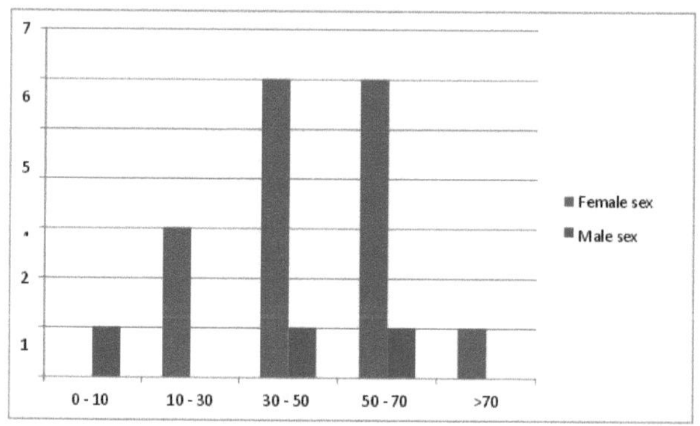


**Figure 3:** Breakdown of patients by age and sex

## 1.5. Site survey

### 1.5.1. Pathological history

We recorded the personal and family history of each patient. Ten patients had pathological histories, including one with type 2 diabetes associated with hypertension (Table I).

**Table II:** Pathological history of patients in our study :

| Personal history | Number of cases |
|---|---|
| Plaque psoriasis | 2 |
| Type 2 diabetes | 1 |
| Hypertension | 3 |
| Celiac disease | 1 |
| Epilepsy | 1 |
| Mental retardation | 1 |
| Subcutaneous lipoma | 1 |
| Scalp ringworm | 1 |

## 1.5.2. Atopy

Only one patient had a history of allergies. He had allergic rhinitis.

## 1.5.3. Drug hypersensitivity

Any history of drug hypersensitivity was present in a single patient with a maculopapular rash to betalactam antibiotics.

## 2. Clinical study :

## 2.1. Functional and general signs :

General condition was preserved in 18 patients. One patient presented with hypovolaemic shock. Fever over 38°C was noted in 16 of the 19 patients. Arthromyalgia was noted in 3 of 19 cases. Pruritus of variable intensity, appearing at the same time as the disease. was reported in 7 patients (36%).

## 2.2. Skin signs :

### 2.2.1. Average time to onset

The average turnaround time is 5.7 days (ranging from one to 21 days).

### 2.2.2. Clinical aspect of acute exanthematic pustulosis :

In our patients, the clinical presentation was characterised by the abrupt onset of a diffuse oedematous sheet erythema, rapidly (within a few hours or days) covered by a cluster of innumerable superficial, sterile, non-follicular pustules less than 5mm in diameter, predominating on the trunk and axillary and inguinal folds.Cutaneous involvement was isolated in 13 patients and mucosal in 6 patients (4 cases of cheilitis, one erosion of the tongue and one genital ulceration). Post-pustular desquamation was observed in one case.

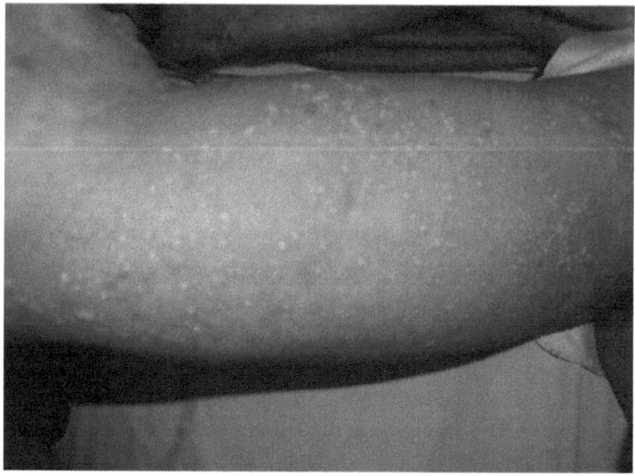

**Figure 4:** Extensive erythematous-edematous and pustular rash (case n°11)

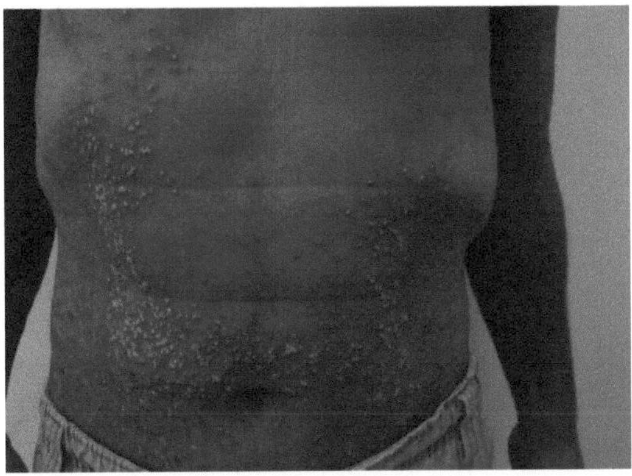

**Figure 5:** Erythemato-oedematous plaques dotted with multiple Non-follicular pustules (case 5)

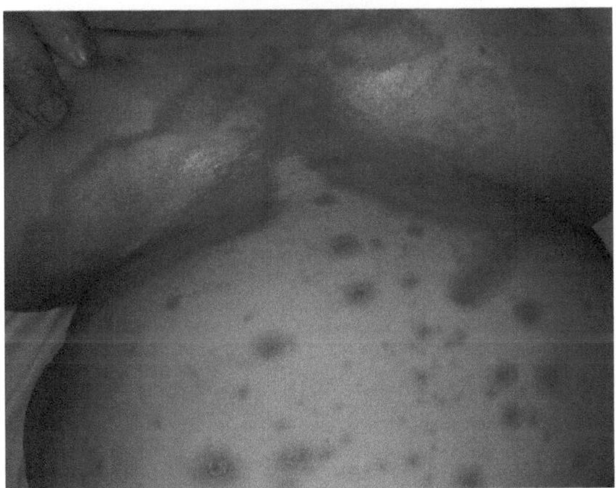

**Figure 6: Erythematous folds with peripheral pustules and cocardiform lesions on the trunk (case 8).**

## 2.2.3. Location of lesions :

The distribution of the erythematous-pustular rash was typical in all cases. Palmoplantar involvement was observed in only one case. Involvement of the face was noted in two cases.

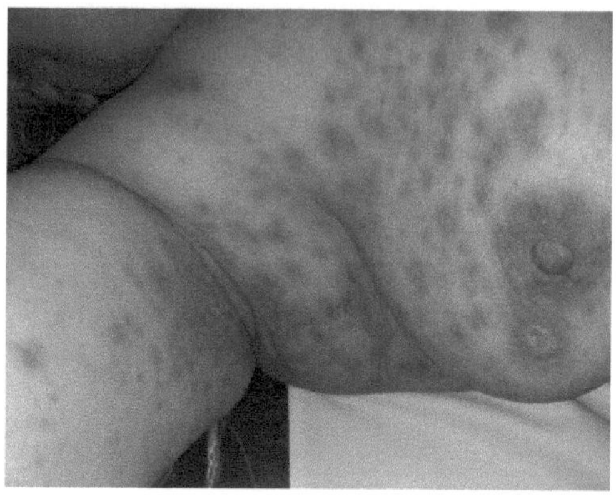

**Figure 7:** Preferential involvement of the major folds (case 8)

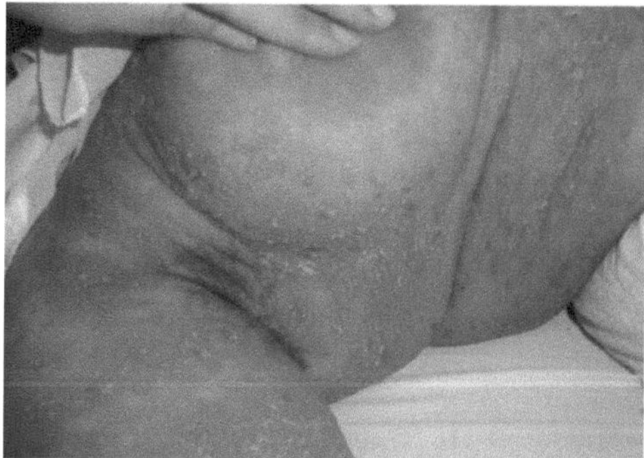

**Figure 8:** Pustular erythematous plaques of the armpits (Case 2)

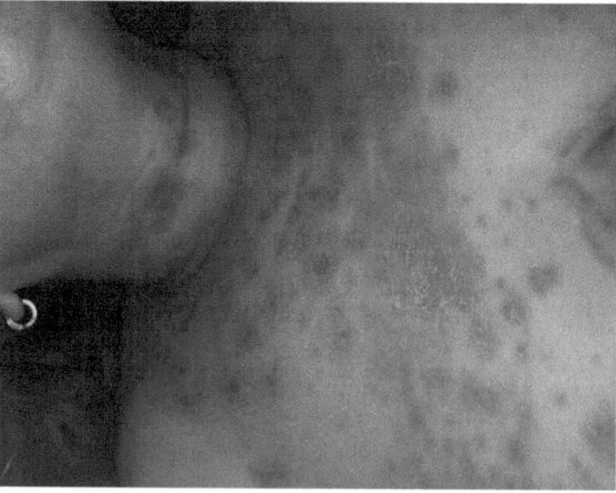

**Figure 9:** Erythematous plaques of the neck and décolleté (case 6)

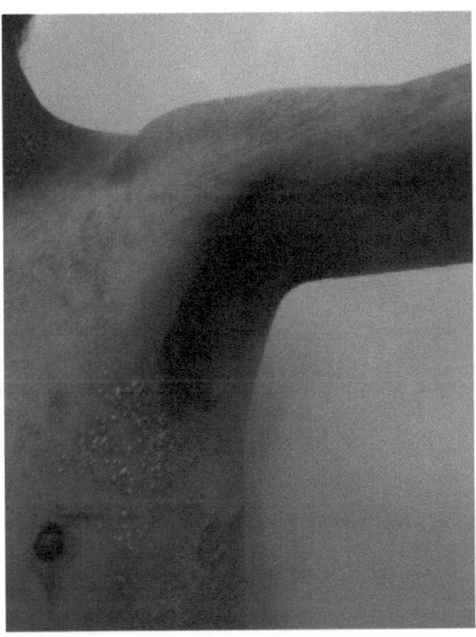

**Figure 10:** Pustular erythematous plaques of the armpits (case 5)

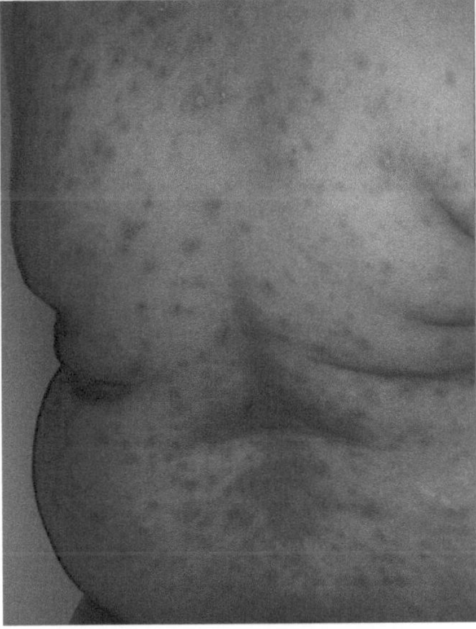

**Figure 11:** Large erythematous plaques on the trunk (case 4)

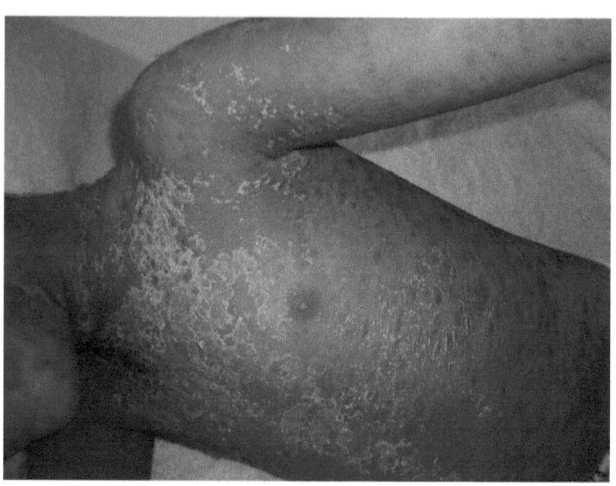

**Figure 12: Diffuse erythematous plaques of the trunk surmounted by a desquamation (case 10)**

**Table III: Location of erythematous and pustular plaques in our patients**

| Appearance of pustules and erythema | Number of cases | Percentage (%) |
|---|---|---|
| Typical | 19 | 100 |
| Distribution of erythematous-pustular plaques | | |
| Broadcast | 19 | 100 |
| Trunk and limbs | 18 | 94 |
| Large folds | 19 | 100 |
| Face | 2 | 10 |
| Palms and soles | 1 | 5 |

## 2.3. Mucosal involvement :

Mucosal involvement was observed in 6 patients (4 cases of cheilitis, tongue erosion in two cases and genital ulceration in one patient).

## 2.4. Systemic involvement :

Cervical adenopathy was present in two cases. One case of hypovolaemic shock was noted in one patient.

## 3. Additional tests:

### 3.1. Biological check-up

### 3.1.1. Blood count

A complete blood count (CBC) was performed in 18 patients and white blood cells ranged from 5,700 to 30,300 cells/mm$^3$ . In 13 patients (68% of cases), neutrophil hyperleukocytosis in excess of 7,000 neutrophils/mm$^3$ was noted. This hyperleukocytosis was associated with hypereosinophilia greater than 500 elements/mm$^3$ in 8 cases (42%).

### 3.1.2. Liver and kidney tests

Liver function tests were carried out in 17 cases and showed no cytolysis. or cholestasis. A renal work-up was carried out in 17 cases and no patient presented with a renal impairment. a disruption of the latter.

### 3.2. Radiological check-up

Chest X-rays were taken in all patients, but the following were not performed did not reveal any pleurisy.

## 4. Chronology of lesion appearance in relation to drug intake :

The onset of skin lesions varied from one to 21 days.

## 5. Drugs implicated in the genesis of PEAG :

The main drugs incriminated in the genesis of acute generalised exanthematous pustulosis were paracetamol in 6 cases, terbinafine in 4 cases, antibiotics in 2 cases, an anti-epileptic drug in 1 case, and an antidepressant in 1 case. 3 cases followed by antihistamines (antiH2) in 1 case and muscle relaxants in 1 case and hydroxyzine in 1 case.

**Table IV:** Drugs implicated in acute generalised exanthematous pustulosis in our patients

| Offending drug | Number of cases |
|---|---|
| Paracetamol | 6 cases |
| Terbinafine | 4 cases |
| Antibiotics | 2 cases |
| Amoxicillin | 1 case |
| Pristinamycin | 1 case |
| Antiepileptics | 3 cases |
| Benzodiazepine | 1 case |
| CARBAMAZEPINE | 2 cases |
| A muscle relaxant | 1 case |
| An anti H2 | 1 case |
| Hydroxyzine | 1 case |

One of our patients had PEAG secondary to a spider bite.

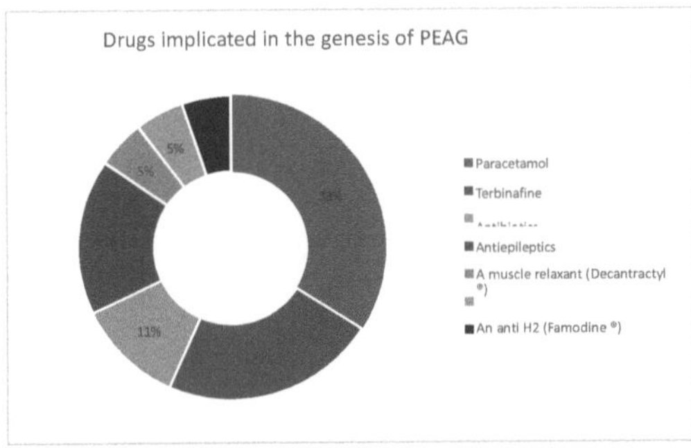


**Figure 13: Drugs implicated in the genesis of PEAG**

## 6. Histopathological examination :

Skin biopsy was performed in 18 cases (94%). The histological aspects were in favour of PEAG in all cases. This examination revealed intra-epidermal and/or sub-corneal pustules, often multilocular and spongiform, associated with oedema of the dermal papilla with an infiltrate of neutrophils and, less consistently, eosinophils (half the patients). These aspects are shown and detailed in Figures 14 and 15.

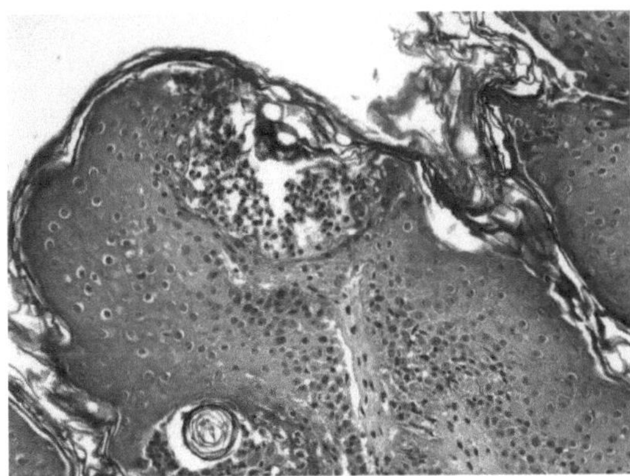

**Figure 14:** Intraepidermal pustules with neutrophils and eosinophils (HEX100)

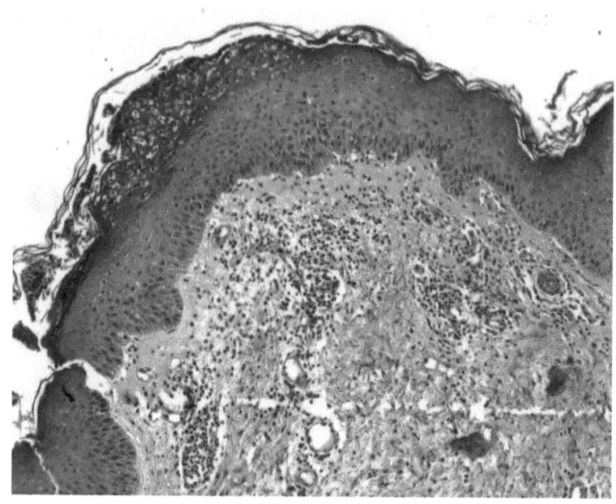

**Figure 15:** Intraepidermal multilocular pustule. The superficial dermis contains a moderate perivascular infiltrate of lymphocytes and eosinophils (HE x100).

## 7. Pharmacovigilance investigation and imputability score :

In our patients, the Bégaud score ranged from I3 probable in 10 patients to I4 very probable in 9 patients.

## 8. Allergological investigations :

In our series, only one patient had patch tests with medication (reactivity to Terbinafine). No patient had an oral provocation test.

## 9. Treatment :

This table summarises the treatments taken by our patients in our series.

**Table V:** Treatments received by patients

| Treatment received | Number of patients |
|---|---|
| General corticosteroid therapy and dermocorticoids | 2 patients |
| Soothing creams and dermocorticoids | 7 patients |
| Antiseptics and dermocorticoids | 6 patients |
| Antihistamines and dermocorticoids | 5 patients |

## 10. Evolution :

All our patients initially progressed well with local and/or general treatment within an average of 7 days. However, 3 patients relapsed and progressed to generalised pustular psoriasis after a delay of one to two months. One of these patients did not undergo a pharmacovigilance investigation. In our series, 16 patients consulted from the 1st episode and 3 patients consulted during the 2nd episode of PEAG. Our patients recovered without sequelae.

# 11. Summary table :

**Table VI:** Summary table of all observations

| Patient | Age (years) | Gender | Episode of PEAG | Deadline onset of the rash | EuroSCAR | Offending drug | Score imputability (Bégaud et al) |
|---|---|---|---|---|---|---|---|
| 1 | 28 | F | 1er | 4 j | 10 | Paracetamol | I3 |
| 2 | 56 | F | 1er | 15 | 9 | Terbinafine | I4 |
| 3 | 27 | F | 1er | 4 | 11 | Atarax | I3 |
| 4 | 54 | H | 1st | 2 | 10 | Pyostacin | I4 |
| 5 | 48 | H | 1st | 2 | 11 | Aspegic/Paracetamol | I3 |
| 6 | 51 | F | 1st | 4 | 10 | Amoxicillin | I4 |
| 7 | 31 | F | 2nd | 5 | 10 | Carbamazepine | I4 |
| 8 | 49 | F | 1st | 1 | 11 | Spider bite | I3 |
| 9 | 56 | F | 1st |  | 10 | Paracetamol | I4 |
| 10 | 7 | H | 1st | 6 | 9 | Terbinafine | I4 |
| 11 | 52 | F | 1st | 20 | 12 | Terbinafine | I4 |
| 12 | 44 | F | 2nd | 1 | 11 | Paracetamol | I4 |
| 13 | 42 | F | 1st | 21 | 9 | Famodine | I3 |
| 14 | 39 | F | 1st | 4 | 8 | Carbamazepine | I3 |
| 15 | 21 | F | 1st | 2 | 9 | Paracetamol | I3 |
| 16 | 85 | F | 1st | 6 | 9 | Paracetamol | I4 |
| 17 | 58 | H | 2nd | 3 | 12 | Decontractyl | I3 |
| 18 | 55 | F | 1st | 7 | 9 | Terbinafine | I3 |
| 19 | 48 | F | 1st | 3 | 18 | Clobazam | I3 |

# DISCUSSION

## 1. Reviews of our study :

Our study reports on the main clinical features of acute generalised exanthematous pustulosis, a rare and severe toxidermia. It can affect both men and women, adults and children. In our series, the drugs incriminated in the genesis of acute generalised exanthematous pustulosis were essentially antibiotics and paracetamol. This toxidermia must be differentiated from other dermatoses that can lead to the appearance of pustules, such as generalised pustular psoriasis and pustular vasculitis, as well as toxidermia with a severe prognosis, such as drug hypersensitivity syndrome (DRESS), Lyell's syndrome and toxic epidermal necrolysis. The limitations of our study were essentially the small number of patients (19), explained by the rarity of this type of toxidermia, and the fact that patch tests were not performed systematically.

## 2. Epidemiology :

### 2.1. Impact :

### 2.1.1. Incidence worldwide :

Little is known about the incidence of PEAG worldwide. It is thought to be underestimated, given the rapid resolution of this dermatosis. Machet et al [21] report an incidence of 1 to 5 cases per million inhabitants per year. This was also confirmed in the Sidoroff study in 2012 [22]. According to Barbaud et al [23], PEAG accounts for 1% of toxidermia. A study carried out at the Fez University Hospital between 2008 and 2013 found that PEAG accounts for 4.1% of all toxidermia.

## 2.1.2. Incidence in Tunisia :

In Tunisia, the incidence of PEAG is not well known. According to a retrospective study carried out in the dermatology department of Habib Thameur Hospital over a two-year period between 2002 and 2004, it accounts for 14.3% of all toxidermia [24]. This figure was confirmed by another study carried out in the dermatology department of La Rabta Hospital in Tunis by Kort et al [21] over a period of 15 years between 1992 and 2007, which estimated the frequency of PEAG at 14.6% of all toxidermia.

## 2.2. Age :

PEAG can affect all age groups, with a predominance of young adults. The mean age of our patients was 44.7 years. Almost 1/3 of patients (6/19) were aged between 30 and 50. However, all ages were affected, from children (a seven-year-old child in our series) to the elderly (an 85-year-old patient in our series). In the literature, PEAG rarely affects children [22,23]. In the Tunisian study by Kort et al, the mean age was close to ours. It was 40.9 years, with extremes ranging from 19 to 81 years [21].

## 2.3. Genre :

In our series, the M/F sex ratio was 0.26. This is in line with several studies which have demonstrated a clear predominance of women in the course of PEAG [6,8,24-26]. Indeed, according to some authors, the frequency may be as high as three women for every man [25]. This predominance could be explained by several factors, in particular hormonal factors (oestrogens are thought to play an immunostimulant role).

## 2.4. Site survey :

### 2.4.1. Atopy :

Only one patient had a history of allergies. He had allergic rhinitis. In the various series in the literature, associations with atopic pathologies are rarely reported during PEAG [21]. Four cases out of 22 were reported in the series by Mebazaa [27].

### 2.4.2. Drug hypersensitivity :

Any history of drug hypersensitivity was present in only one patient in our series.The notion of previous drug hypersensitivity in patients with PEAG has already been reported in the literature, with proportions varying widely from one study to another. In the series by Chang et al [7], 38% of patients had a history of drug hypersensitivity and none in the series by Guevara-Gutierrez [28]. In the series by Mebazaa et al, the percentage was 9%.

## 3. Pathogenesis of PEAG

### 3.1. Pathophysiology of PEAG :

It is reaction immunological reaction (type IV of the Gell and Coombs classification), mediated by T lymphocytes and PNNs. After taking a drug, antigen-presenting cells activate T lymphocytes by presenting the drug molecule in the lymph node (stage 1). The T lymphocytes then multiply and migrate into the skin (stage 2), where they are recruited from the dermis and epidermis (stage 3). They then migrate specifically to the epidermis, where the keratinocytes are killed by the T cells. predominantly CD8, as well as CD4 [29]. Mechanisms are then observed including perforin and granzyme B preformed in the granules of T lymphocytes and natural killers, and to a variable degree, Fas-ligand type reactions (stage 4) [29-32]. This cellular destruction progressively leads to tissue destruction and the formation of subhorn vesicles (stage 5), which are initially filled with T lymphocytes (mainly CD4). These lymphocytes secrete IL-8, GM-CSF and other cytokines, attracting neutrophils and sometimes eosinophils through the dermis to the epidermis (stage 6). Neutrophils fill the vesicles, transforming them into pustules (stage 7) [11,23,33].

## 3.2. Genetic predisposition factors :

A genetic predisposition has been suggested, with a significant increase in certain HLA class I antigens (HLA-B51 phenotype) and certain HLA class II antigens (HLA-DR 11 and HLA- DQ3 phenotypes) [34]. However, there does not appear to be any link between the type of drug responsible for PEAG and the HLA phenotype [35]. In addition, several authors have suggested that mutation of the gene encoding the IL-36 receptor antagonist (IL36Ra), already described in PPG, may predispose individuals to develop PEAG, given the clinical and histological similarities between the two conditions [36-37]. However, larger-scale studies are needed to identify other signalling pathways that could be involved in determining this condition.

## 4. Clinical study :

## 4.1. Clinical aspect :

The clinical picture was typical in all cases, with the sudden onset of an erythemato-oedematopustular rash associated with fever in 13 cases. Fever was generally present and high, ranging from 38°C to 40°C [8,13,30]. In some cases, it may be absent on examination [23]. Pruritus was noted in 7 cases. The presence of pruritus is fairly typical and has often been reported in the majority of study series [14,24,38]. Arthromyalgia was observed in 3 cases, cervical adenopathy in 2 cases, facial oedema in 1 case and shock in 1 case. The general condition is often well preserved during PEAG [4,9,13,24]. However, cases of PEAG with a very altered state have been reported [39- 40], with even cases of death in extreme situations [28]. In the study by Kort et al [21], 14 patients (63.6%) had a fever of more than 38°C and one of them had an altered general condition requiring hospital treatment in an intensive care unit. Seven patients (31.8%) had pruritus of varying intensity that appeared at the same time as the skin involvement. In the series by Frioui et al [41], bilateral pleurisy was noted in one patient.

## 4.2. Headquarters :

In our series, the most frequent location was the trunk and/or limbs (19 cases). Involvement of the large folds was noted in all cases. This has been confirmed in various series in the literature [7,10,30,42]. Involvement of the face was observed in 2 cases, and of the palms and soles in a single case. No involvement of the scalp was noted. The rash was generalised in all cases. In the series by Alniemi et al [6], the rash was diffuse in 96% of cases and limited to the folds in 4%. In the series studied at the pharmacovigilance centre between 2000 and 2016, the involvement was generalised in 38 cases and localised in two patients [43]. Mucosal involvement was observed in 6 patients, with cheilitis in 4 cases, ulceration of the tongue in two cases and genital ulceration in one case. In the literature, mucosal involvement is observed in around 20% of cases and is generally limited to a single site, the most common being the buccal mucosa [6,7,24,42,44,45]. This involvement is associated with skin involvement and may be oral, with erosive lesions of the mouth, tongue and lips [8,42], or more rarely genital, with erosive lesions [17]. Rare cases of ocular involvement such as conjunctivitis have also been reported in the literature [8,21].

## 4.3. Additional tests :

### 4.3.1. Biology :

Biology revealed neutrophilia in 13 cases and hyper-eosinophilia in 8. According to the EuroSCAR study, neutrophilia is one of the criteria for PEAG [17,32]. Eosinophilia is observed in about a third of cases [3,14,44].

No patient had a disturbance of the renal or hepatic balance. In the Tunisian series by kort et al [21], hepatic cytolysis was present in two cases, hepatic cholestasis in one case and cytolysis associated with hepatic cholestasis in two cases. Functional renal failure was present in two cases. In the series by Frioui et al [41], biological tests revealed neutrophilia in 19 cases, hyper-eosinophilia in 8 cases, hepatic cytolysis in 4 cases and cholestasis in 2 cases.

**4.3.2. Histology :**

Skin biopsy was performed in 18 cases (94%). The histological aspects were in favour of PEAG in all cases. This examination revealed intra-epidermal and/or sub-corneal pustules, often multilocular and spongiform, associated with oedema of the dermal papilla with an infiltrate of neutrophils and, less consistently, eosinophils (half the patients). These results are in line with the data in the literature, in particular the multicentre study by Halevy et al which included 102 cases, making it the largest series to study the different histopathological aspects found in PEAG [44] and the series by Frioui et al [41].

**5. Diagnosis :**

**5.1. Positive diagnosis :**

All cases of PEAG are diagnosed according to the criteria of the EURO-SCAR group. The **EuroSCAR** group's classification is based on clinical, evolutionary and histological criteria, making it easier to differentiate PEAG from clinically and/or histologically similar dermatoses such as pustular psoriasis [3,46]. The diagnosis of PEAG is ruled out if the score is less than or equal to 0, possible if it is between 1 and 4, probable between 5 and 7 and certain between 8 and 12 [4,5]. The most of studies recent on the PEAG have adopted this classification. In our study, using the criteria of the EuroSCAR group, the diagnosis of PEAG was certain in all patients.

## 5.2. Allergological investigations :

If an allergic reaction is suspected, and it is not possible to make a decision on the basis of questioning alone, an allergological evaluation is essential, especially when the drug in question is essential or frequently prescribed, i.e. when avoidance alone is not an option. The provocation test remains the gold standard for aetiological diagnosis, but it is rarely carried out because of its potentially dangerous nature. This justifies the increasing use of skin tests, particularly patch tests.Patch testing in PEAG is a practical diagnostic method for determining the drug responsible. Drug patch tests should be performed on the site previously affected by EPF, especially if several molecules are involved [30,31]. According to the recommendations of the European Society of Contact Dermatitis, patch tests can be performed with the drug in its marketed form, diluted 30% in petroleum jelly. Patch testing could therefore be suggested as a first-line investigation in PEAG, given that it is an easy and often well-tolerated procedure with relatively good sensitivity [9,18,47,48,49]. In our series, only one patient had drug skin tests to identify the suspect drug.

## 5.3. Differential diagnosis :

### 5.3.1. Von Zumbusch's generalized pustular psoriasis (PPG)

This is the main differential diagnosis for PEAG. Table VII below summarises the differences between PEAG and PPG.

**Table VII:** Main criteria for differentiating a PEAG from a PPG [30].

| Criteria | PEAG | PPG |
|---|---|---|
| History of psoriasis | Generally non-existent | Often present |
| Notion of recent medication intake | Very frequent | Less frequent |
| Distribution of lesions | Initially predominant in the folds | More diffuse |
| Size of pustules | Tiny (pinhead | Larger |
| Associated arthritis | Associated arthritis | Approximately 30%. |
| Histology | Keratinocyte necrosis, oedema Papillary dermis, vasculitis, exocytosis of NEPs | Papillomatosis, acanthosis, vessels winding. |
| Recovery time | Rapid (often <15 days) | Longer |

## 5.3.2. Other :

Drug hypersensitivity syndrome or DRESS syndrome, Lyell's syndrome or toxic epidermal necrolysis (TEN) and infectious pustulosis may be a differential diagnosis with PEAG.

## 6.  Treatment and progress :

In our series, in addition to stopping the causative drug, symptomatic treatment was prescribed. Local corticosteroid therapy was prescribed in 19 patients. Anti-H1 drugs were prescribed in 5 patients. Emollients were prescribed in 7 patients. Antiseptic baths were prescribed in 6 patients. General corticosteroid therapy was indicated in 2 patients due to the severity of the clinical picture (prednisone at a dose of 1mg/kg/d for one and 0.5 mg/kg/d for the other, with gradual tapering off). All our patients initially progressed well with local and/or general treatment within an average of 7 days. However, 3 patients relapsed and progressed to generalised pustular psoriasis. In the literature, the course of this toxidermia is often favourable [24,30,50] and recovery is usually obtained in less than 15 days after stopping the drug responsible [17,24,50]. Hospitalisation may be necessary during PEAG depending on the intensity of the fever, the extent of skin lesions, or sometimes systemic complications [9], as in the case of one of our patients who was admitted for shock and two others who were admitted for extensive lesions.

## 7. Drugs responsible for PEAG :

### 7.1. Antibiotics :

In our series, betalactams were incriminated in 6 cases, i.e. 36% of cases, and terbinafine in 4 cases, i.e. 22% of cases. This is not consistent with the data in the literature [5,14,18,42,43], where betalactam antibiotics are the most frequently implicated. In Tunisia, a retrospective descriptive study, conducted at the CNPV between January 2000 and December 2016 [43], PEAG was attributed to antibiotics in 15 patients (42%).In the series by Frioui (29 cases) [41], the aetiological work-up found a medicinal cause in 19 cases, including amoxicillin: 6 cases, oxacillin: 1 case, and pristinamycin: 5 cases. In the series by Chamli et al [51], the pharmacovigilance survey incriminated the role of hydroxychloroquine in 1 case among 8 patients, oxacillin (1 case), amoxicillin (2 cases), clindamycin (1 case) and teicoplanin (1 case). Antibiotics were also incriminated in all patients with PEAG in the study conducted at the Fes pharmacovigilance centre [52].

### 7.2. Other medicines :

### a. Antifungals :

Among the antifungal agents responsible for PEAG, terbinafine tops the list [5,13,18,23,53]. In our patients, it was responsible for 4 cases of PEAG. According to the literature, there are only about thirty reported cases of PEAG induced by terbinafine. It is characterised by a late onset [54].

## b. Paracetamol :

Recent publications increasingly incriminate paracetamol in the occurrence of PEAG [55]. Indeed, 11% of patients included in the series from the pharmacovigilance centre presented a PEAG secondary to paracetamol [43] and 10.3% in the series by Frioui [41]. In our series, 6 patients (31.5%) developed PEAG after taking paracetamol.

## c. Antiepileptics :

Antiepileptic drugs are frequently implicated in the occurrence of SCARs, particularly in DRESS syndrome and, to a lesser extent, in PEAG [18,42]. In the series by Kort et al, carbamazepine was implicated in only one case. In the series by Chang et al [7], carbamazepine and phenytoin were implicated in two cases. In our series, antiepileptic drugs were incriminated in three cases (15.7%), including carbamazepine in two cases and carbazam in a single case.

## d. Other exceptional medicines :

In our series, PEAG was induced by the use of a muscle relaxant (Decontractyl®) in one case, an antiH2 drug (Famodine®) in one case and an antihistamine (Atarax®) in one case. We did not find any cases of PEAG related to these drugs in the literature.

# CONCLUSIONS

Acute generalised exanthematous pustulosis (AGEP) is a rare and serious condition, characterised by the sudden onset of a febrile erythematous-oedematous and pustular rash. This rash is often accompanied by neutrophilic polynucleosis. PEAG can occur at any age, although its onset in children is atypical [9]. The aetiology is drug-induced in over 90% of cases. However, it is sometimes difficult and time-consuming to identify the inducing drug, particularly in patients with multiple medications, especially as other, albeit rare, aetiologies for PEAG have been reported, particularly infectious or post-mercury.The drugs most often responsible are antibiotics such as beta-lactams and pristinamycin [2,3]. PEAG is a model of delayed drug hypersensitivity mediated by CD8 T lymphocytes [3]. The aim of our study was to investigate the epidemiological, clinical, therapeutic and evolutionary characteristics of acute generalised exanthematous pustulosis and to identify the drug classes that most frequently cause this condition, based on a hospital series of 19 cases. We conducted a retrospective, monocentric, descriptive study in the Dermatology Department of the Habib Thameur Hospital in Tunis over 14 years (January 2008-December 2021), recording 19 cases.In our series, the incidence of acute generalised exanthematous pustulosis was estimated at 0.9 cases per 10,000 consultations per year, indicating the rarity of this toxidermia. The average age was 44.7 years. AGEP can affect people of all ages, with a predominance in young adults. Children may also be affected (one case in our series). The sex ratio M/F was 0,26. PEAG mainly affects women. In the various published series, this predominance is frequently found in With the exception of a few series where the sex ratio was close to 1. The diagnosis of PEAG in our patients was based on clinical and paraclinical criteria, validated by the score established in 2001 by the EuroSCAR group. The clinical presentation was typically erythematous and diffuse pustular. Mucosal involvement is rarely observed in PEAG and is often limited to the oral mucosa. Nevertheless, in our series, cheilitis was observed in 4 cases and was associated with ulcerations of the tongue in two cases and of the genitals in one case. The onset of skin lesions varied, ranging from a few hours to a few days after taking the drug. A fever greater than 38°C was noted in 13 patients (68%) and hyperleukocytosis with PNN greater than 7000 elements/mm3 was reported in 13 patients (68%). The main drugs implicated in the genesis of acute generalised exanthematous pustulosis were antibiotics in 12 cases (63.1%), followed by paracetamol in 6 cases.Skin biopsies were taken in 18 patients (94%). The most common features were subcorneal and/or intraepidermal pustules in all cases, associated with oedema of the dermal papilla with an infiltrate of neutrophils and, less consistently, eosinophils (half the patients). The episode of PEAG was inaugural in 16 patients and a recurrence in 3 patients. A pharmacovigilance survey was carried out in all patients. to identify the drug involved and the imputability score intrinsic drug effect ranged from probable I3 in 10 patients to very probable I4 in 9 patients. Only one patient had a patch test identifying the suspect drug. All patients were treated with local corticosteroids combined with general corticosteroids in two cases and antihistamines in 6 cases, with the suspect drug being discontinued, leading to a good clinical outcome. Although rare, PEAG remains an event of great interest in the field of therapeutic safety and the reassessment of the benefit-risk ratio of drugs, like any serious cutaneous event. At the end of this study, we would like to emphasise the importance of a positive diagnosis of PEAG and reiterate the importance of performing a skin biopsy in order to obtain a definitive diagnosis. We must also stress the importance of aetiological diagnosis, which relies firstly on rigorous questioning and secondly on skin tests, particularly patch tests. Patch tests have proved their worth in distinguishing between different suspected drugs. They should therefore be an integral part of the diagnostic process for AEGD.

## REFERENCES

1. Baker H, Ryan TJ. Generalized pustular psoriasis. A clinical and epidemiological study of 104 cases. Br J Dermatol. 1968 Dec;80(12):771- 93.

2. Beylot C, Bioulac P, Doutre MS. Acute generalized exanthematic pustulosis (four cases). Ann DermatolVenereol. 1980 Jan;107(1):37-48.

3. Roujeau JC, Bioulac-Sage P, Bourseau C, Guillaume JC, Bernard P, Lok C, et al.Acute generalized exanthematous pustulosis. Analysis of 63 cases. Arch Dermatol. 1991 Sep;127(9):1333-8.

4. Sidoroff A, Halevy S, Bavinck JN, Vaillant L, Roujeau JC. Acute generalized exanthematous pustulosis (AGEP) a clinical reaction pattern. J CutanPathol. 2001 Mar;28(3):113-9.

5. Sidoroff A, Dunant A, Viboud C, Halevy S, Bavinck JN, Naldi L, et al. Risk factors for acute generalized exanthematous pustulosis (AGEP)- results of a multinational case-control study (EuroSCAR). Br J Dermatol. 2007 Nov;157(5):989-96.

6. Alniemi DT, Wetter DA, Bridges AG, El Azhary RA, Davis MD, Camilleri MJ, et al. Acute generalized exanthematou spustulosis: clinical characteristics, etiologic associations, treatments, and outcomes in a series of 28 patients at Mayo clinic,1996-2013. Int J Dermatol. 2017 Apr;56(4):405-14.

7. Chang SL, Huang YH, Yang CH, Hu S, Hong HS. Clinical manifestations and characteristics of patients with acute generalized exanthematous pustulosis in Asia. Acta Derm Venereol. 2008 Mar;88(4):363-5.

8. Choi MJ, Kim HS, Park HJ, Park CJ, Lee JD, Lee JY, et al. Clinicopathologic manifestations of 36 Korean patients with acute generalized exanthematou spustulosis: a case series and review of the literature. Ann Dermatol. 2010 May;22(2):163-9.

9. Hotz C, Valeyrie Allanore L, Haddad C, Bouvresse S, Ortonne N, Duong TA, et al. Systemic involvement of acute generalized exanthematous pustulosis: a retrospective study on 58 patients. Br J Dermatol. 2013 Dec;169(6):1223-32.

10. Thienvibul C, Vachiramon V, Chanprapaph K. Five-year retrospective review of acute generalized exanthematous pustulosis. Dermatol Res Pract. 2015 Dec;2015:260928.

11. Hoetzenecker W, Nageli M, Mehra ET, Jensen AN, Saulite I, Schmid GrendelmeierP, et al. Adverse cutaneous drug eruptions: current understanding. Semin Immunopathol. 2016 Jan;38(1):75-86.

12. Moreno Arrones OM, CarrilloGijon R, Sendagorta E, RiosBuceta L. Acute generalized exanthematous pustulosis simulating Stevens-Johnson syndrome/toxic epidermal necrolysis associated with the use of vismodegib. JAAD Case Rep. 2018 Jan;4(2):123-5.

13. Peermohamed S, Haber RM. Acute generalized exanthematous pustulosis simulating toxic epidermal necrolysis: a case report and review of the literature. Arch Dermatol. 2011 Jun;147(6):697-701.

14. Kostopoulos TC, Krishna SM, Brinster NK, OrtegaLoayza AG. Acute generalized exanthematous pustulosis: atypical presentations and outcomes. J EurAcad Dermatol Venereol. 2015 Feb;29(2):209-14.

15. Szatkowski J, Schwartz RA. Acute generalized exanthematous pustulosis(AGEP): a review and update. J Am AcadDermatol. 2015 Nov;73(5):843-8.

16. Bégaud B, Evreux JC, Jouglard J, Lagier G. Imputability of unexpected or toxic effects of drugs. Update of the method used in France. Therapie. Mar 1985;40(2):111-8.

17. Machet L, Martin L, Vaillant L. Acute generalised exanthematous pustulosis. Ann Dermatol Venereol. 2001 Jan;128(1):73-9.

18. Sidoroff A. Acute generalized exanthematous pustulosis. Chem Immunol Allergy. 2012May;97:139-48.

19. Barbaud A, Reichertpenetrat S, Trechot P, Jacquin Petit MA, Ehlinger A, Noirez V, et al. The use of skin testing in the investigation of cutaneous adverse drug reactions. Br J Dermatol. 1998 Jul;139(1):49-58.

20. Souissi A. Les réactions cutanées aux médicaments à propos d'une série hospitalière de 28 cas [dissertation: medicine]. Tunis: Université de Tunis El Manar; 2005.

21. Kort R. La pustulose exanthématique aigue généralisée : étude de 22 cas [mémoire : médecine]. Tunis: University of Tunis El Manar; 2008.

22. Bonnetblanc JM. Cutaneous drug reactions in children.

Ann Dermatol Venereol. Dec 1997;124(4):339-45.

23. Ersoy S, Paller AS, Mancini AJ. Acute generalized exanthematous pustulosis in children. Arch Dermatol. 2004 Sep;140(9):1172-3.

24. Fernando SL. Acute generalized exanthematous pustulosis. Australas J Dermatol. 2012 May;53(2):87-92.

25. Choon SE, Der YS, Lai NL, Yu SE, Yap XL, Nalini NM. Clinical characteristics, culprit drugs and outcome of patients with acute generalized exanthematous pustulosis seen in Hospital Sultanah Aminah, Johor Bahru. Med J Malaysia. 2018 Aug;73(4):220-5.

26. De A, Das S, Sarda A, Pal D, Biswas P. Acute generalized exanthematous pustulosis: an update. Indian J Dermatol. 2018 Jan;63(1):22-9.

27. Mebazaa A, kort R, Zaiem A, Elleuch D. Acute generalized exanthematous pustulosis: study of 22 cases. Rev La tunisie medicale. 2010 December.88(12):910_5

28. Guevara Gutierrez E, Uribejimenez E, Diazcanchola M, Tlacuiloparra A. Acute generalized exanthematous pustulosis: report of 12 cases and literature review.Int J Dermatol. 2009 Mar;48(3):253-8.

29. Speeckaert MM, Speeckaert R, Lambert J, Brochez L. Acute generalized exanthematou spustulosis: an overview of the clinical,

immunological and diagnostic concepts. Eur J Dermatol. 2010 Jul;20(4):425-33.

30. Feldmeyer L, Heidemeyer K, Yawalkar N. Acute generalized exanthematous pustulosis: pathogenesis, genetic background, clinical variants and therapy. Int J Mol Sci. 2016 Jul;17(8):1214.

31. Schlapbach C, Zawodniak A, Irla N, Adam J, Hunger RE, Yerly D, et al. NKp46+cells express granulysin in multiple cutaneous adverse drug reactions. Allergy. 2011 Nov;66(11):1469-76.

32. Schmid S, Kuechler PC, Britschgi M, Steiner UC, Yawalkar N, Limat A, et al. Acute generalized exanthematous pustulosis: role of cytotoxic T cells in pustule formation. Am J Pathol. 2002 Dec;161(6):2079-86.

33. Mashiah J, Brenner S. A systemic reaction to patch testing for the evaluation of acute generalized exanthematous pustulosis. Arch Dermatol. 2003 Sep;139(9):1181-3.

34. Bernard PH, Lizieuxparneix V, Miossec V. HLA and genetic predisposition in acute generalized exanthematous pustulosis (AGEP) and maculopapular exanthema (MPE). Ann Dermatol Venereol. Mar 1995;122:38-9.

35. McCormack M, Alfirevic A, Bourgeois S, Farrell JJ, Kasperaviciute D, CarringtonM, et al. HLA-A*3101 and carbamazepine-induced hypersensitivity reactions in europeans. N Engl J Med. 2011 Mar;364(12):1134-43.

36. Li X, Chen M, Fu X, Zhang Q, Wang Z, Yu G, et al. Mutation analysis of theIL36RN gene in Chinese patients with generalized pustular psoriasis with/without psoriasis vulgaris. J Dermatol Sci. 2014 Nov;76(2):132-8.

37. Nakai N, Sugiura K, Akiyama M, Katoh N. Acute generalized exanthematous pustulosis caused by dihydrocodeine phosphate in a patient with psoriasis vulgaris and a heterozygous IL36RN mutation. JAMA Dermatol. 2015 Mar;151(3):311-5.

38. Adler NR, Aung AK, Ergen EN, Trubiano J, Goh MS, Phillips EJ. Recent advances in the understanding of severe cutaneous adverse reactions. Br J Dermatol. 2017 Nov;177(5):1234-47.

39. Moling O, Perino F, Piccin A. Acute generalized exanthematous pustulosis withoverlap features of toxic epidermal necrolysis/Stevens- Johnson syndrome. Int J Dermatol. 2014 Jan;53(1):27-8.

40. Leclair MA, Maynard B, Saint Pierre C. Acute generalized exanthematous spustulosis with severe organ dysfunction. Can Med Assoc J. 2009

Sep;181(6):393-6.

41. Frioui R, Amina A, Tabka M, Jouini W, Mokni S. Acute generalized exanthematous pustulosis: a hospital series of 29 cases. Rev Med interne. Sept 2021;42:206.

42. Teo YX, Walsh SA. Severe adverse drug reactions. Clin Med. 2016 Feb;16(1):79-83.

43. Harbaoui S. La pustulose exanthématique aigue généralisée: diagnostic clinique et imputabilité médicamenteuse [dissertation: medicine]. Tunis: University of Tunis El Manar; 2019.

44. Halevy S, Kardaun SH, Davidovicci B, Wechsler J. The spectrum ofhistopathological features in acute generalized exanthematous pustulosis: astudy of 102 cases. Br J Dermatol. 2010 Dec;163(6):1245-52.

45. Vigarios E, Tournier E, Pouessel D, Cohen E, Sibaud V. Oral lesions of acutegeneralized exanthematouspustulosis. Int J Dermatol. 2017 Dec;56(12):1465-7.

46. Defo D, Martin L, Esteve E, Padonou F. Acute generalized exanthematous pustulosis: a study of 22 cases. Ann Dermatol Venereol. May 2007;134:33-4.

47. Syrigou E, Grapsa D, Charpidou A, Syrigos K. Acute generalized exanthematous pustulosis Induced by amoxicillin/clavulanic acid: Report of a case presenting with generalized lymphadenopathy. J Cutan Med Surg. 2015 Nov;19(6):592-4.

48. Barbaud A, Collet E, Milpied B, Assier H, Staumont D, Avenel Audran M, et al. A multicenter study to determine the value and safety of drug patch tests for the three main classes of severe cutaneous adverse drug reactions. Br J Dermatol. 2013 Mar;168(3):555-62.

49. Walsh S, Creamer D. A diagnostic challenge: acute generalized exanthematous pustulosis or pustular psoriasis due to terbinafine: comment. Clin Exp Dermatol. 2012 Dec;37(8):919.

50. Cho YT, Chu CY. Treatments for severe cutaneous adverse reactions. J

Immunol Res. 2017 Dec;2017:1503709.

51. Chamli A, Litaiem N, Khammouma F, Karray M. Acute generalized exanthematous pustulosis: a series of 8 cases. Rev Med Interne. Oct 2021;42:199-206.

52. Ross CL, Shevchenko A, Mollanazar NK, Hsu S, Motaparthi K. Acute generalized exanthematous pustulosis due to terbinafine. Dermatol Ther. 2018 Jul;31(4):e12617.

53. Gara S, Zaouak A, Hammami H, Fenniche S. Terbinafine-induced acute generalised exanthematous pustulosis. Rev Med Interne. Oct 2021;42:95-206.

54. Boccaletti V, Cortelazzi C, Fantini C, Tognetti E, Fabrizi G, Pagliarello C, et al. Acute generalized exanthematous pustulosis following paracetamol ingestion in a child. Pediatr Allergy Immunol. 2015 Jun;26(4):391-2.

55. Ingen-Housz-Oro S, Duong TA, De Prost N, Colin A, Fardet L, Lebrun Vignes B and al. Treatment of  toxidermiaAnn DermatolVenereol.2018;145(6):454-67.

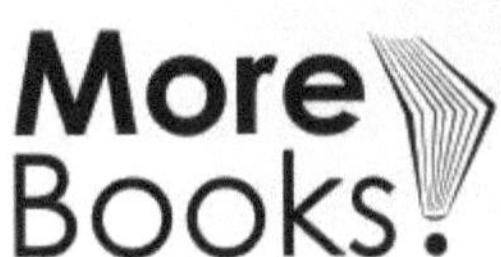
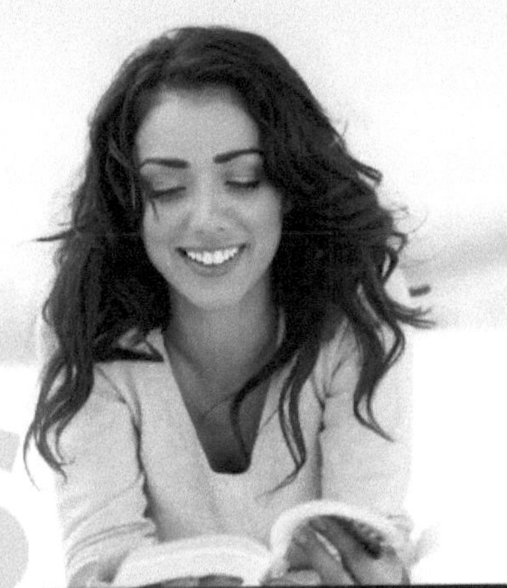

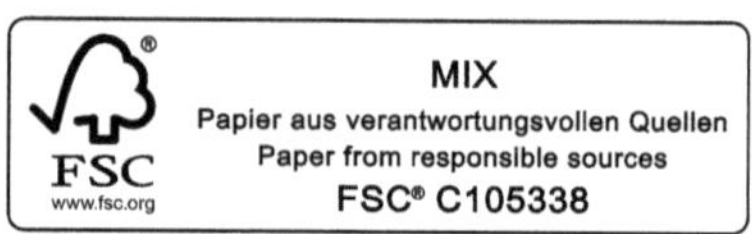


Printed by Books on Demand GmbH, Norderstedt / Germany